# KITCHEN COSMETICS

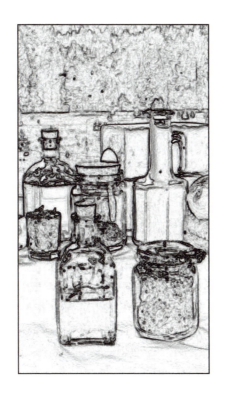

Published by 3norns press
Box 144
Crescent Valley
British Columbia
Canada
V0G 1H0

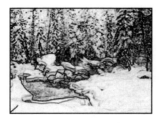

Printed and bound in Canada.
Photography by Dan Norn
Edited by Julia Garry

National Library of Canada Cataloguing
in Publication Data

Norn, Jan, 1936-
 Kitchen cosmetics
 Includes index.
 ISBN  0-9731099-0-4
 1.   Skin care and hygiene. 2. Cosmetics.
 3.Toilet preparations.
     1.Garry, Julia, 1965- 11. Title.
RA778.N67.2002  646.7'26  C2002-910703-2

# KITCHEN COSMETICS

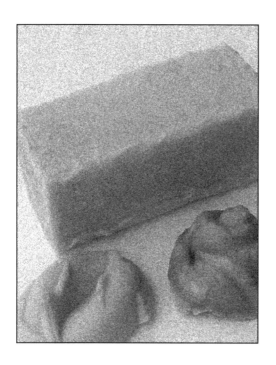

## DO-IT-YOURSELF SKIN CARE

## JAN NORN

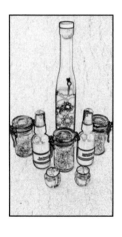

# INDEX

# INTRODUCTION

◆ ◆ ◆

Since the dawn of time, women have loved cosmetics. Be it bear-grease and woad or complex creams and lotions, grooming has always been an attribute of the human female.

Somewhere during the last century, cosmetics stopped being something made from recipes handed down from mother to daughter and became a huge and competitive industry, presided over by people intent on making as much money as possible. Commercial advertising happened to us and 'beauty' became very costly (in some cases to our health as well as to our wallets).

Cosmetics are now manufactured from a huge variety of materials, from herbal oils and essences to salts, solvents, silicas, hormones, polymers, petroleum and a bewilderment of intricate chemical compounds. It used to be believed that the skin formed a barrier that prevented the things we put on it from penetrating any further. We now know that "what goes on goes in" and that unhealthy ingredients on the outside can eventually lead to trouble on the inside.

In her book, "Beauty to Die For", Judi Vance describes her love of cosmetics, her years of unidentifiable illness and the long slow process of repairing and cleansing her immune system. She includes a fascinating list of common cosmetic ingredients and their effects. If you care about your skin, read this list! And start reading labels on your cosmetics.

Dr. Samuel Epstein, founder of the Cancer Prevention Society, has compiled "The Safe Shopper's Bible" which lists many household items, including cosmetics, in respect to their cancer-causing potential. Lots of surprises in this book, too.

I have been making my own cosmetics for the past three decades, but after reading about the effects of some of the ingredients that I had always considered safe and beneficial, I reformulated all of my recipes. Old favourites like lanolin, talc, borax and petroleum jelly no longer have a place in my cupboard, having been replaced by such things as emu oil, slippery elm, honey or beeswax.

Because I know exactly what goes into my recipes, and because I store them in the fridge (most recipes can be frozen) instead of loading them with preservatives, I know that they have no ill effects on my immune system and that they will benefit my skin and hair. Cosmetic cookery is no more difficult than the conventional kind. It will save you a great deal of money and will give you hours of fun, along with the satisfaction of knowing that you did it yourself.

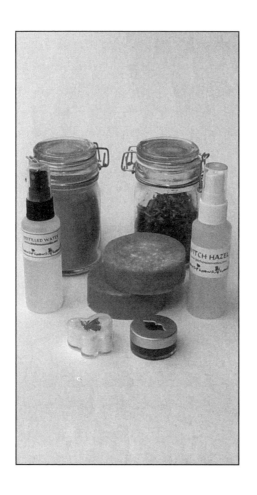

# CARING FOR YOUR FACE

❖  ❖  ❖

*Photo:  Volcanic clay, wild sage, distilled water, goat's milk soap,*
*witch hazel, emu oil cream, dry skin mask.*

# HOW TO WASH YOUR FACE!

◆ ◆ ◆

Don't be silly, you say - I've been doing this all my life. Well, so had I, but it took me 54 years to figure out the right way. My life has always been busy, so a quick kitty-lick with warm water morning and night was about all the attention my face received. If I had been wearing make-up, I would cream it off with any available cleanser and wash gently with water, but never with soap. Soap made my skin feel tight and shiny. I know why about 90% of the women I talk to say, "I can't use soap on my face."

It was not until I started making my own soap that I realized the huge difference between homemade and commercial. At that point I started washing my face with soap from <u>my</u> kitchen and realized that I had been missing something for about half a century.

Now think about it. Would you wash your clothes in oil (even good quality oil) mixed with detergent, then wipe them off and expect them to be clean? So how about cleaning your face the same way? Not the best plan.

Skin is constantly renewing itself by sloughing off dead cells and excreting oil. It also gets dirty. It needs to be cleaned thoroughly and firmly, not just patted at with cleanser. After cleaning, it must be PH balanced, hydrated and moisturised.

- Pure unscented goat's milk soap or pure vegetable soap

- A piece of loofah or a good cotton face cloth

- Witch hazel in a spray mister

- Distilled water in a spray mister

- Moisturising cream

1. If you are wearing heavy makeup, remove with a natural cleansing cream (page 15), particularly around the delicate eye areas. Remove with cotton, not tissues.

2. Wash thoroughly with soap and scrub briskly. Soap does not destroy dirt; it catches the tiny molecules and slides them off your skin. Scrubbing helps to open clogged pores and dislodge clinging molecules. It also stimulates circulation. Be firm with your face!

3. Rinse with clear water and dry.

4. Mist face and neck with witch hazel. Allow to dry naturally.

5. Mist with distilled water. Remember that water is the single most important thing that you can put on your skin. Your body is more than 99% water after all, and your skin craves it.

6. Moisturise with a natural preparation.

◆ ◆ ◆

*Your skin will feel like rose petals.*

# APPLYING CREAM
# TO YOUR FACE

◆ ◆ ◆

No, you don't just grab that pot of cream and scrabble it into your skin!  Slow down and spend a few soothing minutes with this gentle and uplifting exercise.

### YOU WILL NEED

❖ A safe moisturising cream

❖ Clean hands

❖ A little time

1. Always stroke upwards when applying cream.  Avoid stretching your skin down.  Starting at the base of your throat, apply cream with clean fingertips.  Using long, upward strokes, massage in gently from throat to chin, with at least 20 strokes to stimulate circulation.

2. Now use both hands and work from the centre of the chin to your ear lobes - 20 more strokes, please.

3. Starting at the corners of your mouth, draw imaginary pussy-cat whiskers over your cheeks.  Stop when you reach the delicate skin under your eyes, but cover all the surface of your cheeks with another 20 strokes.

4.  Begin at the centre of your upper lip and make 20 short strokes to the corners of your mouth. Still using both hands, start at the outside of your nose, cream upwards between your eyes, and spread towards your temples in a Y shape; 20 again.

5.  Finally, pat cream briskly into the fragile areas below your eyes and on your eyelids.

◆ ◆ ◆

Massaging the cream into your skin not only helps it to penetrate, but stimulates circulation. Extra blood flow helps to carry away impurities and promotes healing.

If you are concerned about being allergic to any of the ingredients used in the recipes on the following pages, do the simple allergy test on page 56. If the ingredient upsets your skin, replace it with something similar that does not cause you problems.

**N O T E S**

*For the fun of it, count the number of personal care products you use every morning before going to work.*

*Do the same for the evening. If there is a man in your family, how many does he use?*

*Now add up what they all cost. Surprised? You can make your own safe products for much less.*

# CLEANSING CREAM

◆  ◆  ◆

Milk was Cleopatra's beauty secret.  She took baths in it.
We think that yoghurt is even better, not for baths but for
a gentle cleanser, full of natural enzymes and rich
creamy milk.

### INGREDIENTS

- ◆  4 tablespoons plain yoghurt

- ◆  1 teaspoon fresh pineapple juice

- ◆  1/2 teaspoon witch hazel.

Add juice and witch hazel to yoghurt and stir in gently
with plastic spoon or spatula.  Do not heat.  Spoon into
jar and keep refrigerated when not in use.  Best made in
small quantities and used within expiry date of yoghurt.

◆  ◆  ◆

### TO USE

1.  Apply liberally, starting at the neck area and working
    up.  Follow the same pattern that you use to apply
    moisturiser (page 13) always working with upward
    strokes.

2. Remove with cotton pads or a damp cotton facecloth. Never use tissues on your face. They may be sanitary, but they are made of wood processed with a lot of chemicals.

3. Finish by washing your face (page 10).

## WHY?

❖ **Yoghurt** because it removes make-up and impurities gently and effectively, while actually nourishing the skin.

❖ **Pineapple Juice** contains bromelain, which helps to soften and exfoliate dead skin cells.

❖ **Witch Hazel** stimulates circulation and restores PH balance.

## NOTES
*When a harmful substance is swallowed, your digestive system may be able to cope with it.*

*But when something harmful is absorbed through your skin, it goes directly into the blood stream.*

# MASK FOR DRY SKIN

◆ ◆ ◆

A clay mask is an instant revitalizer for dull, tired skin. As the clay dries, it tightens the skin and stimulates circulation. An enforced half hour or so of complete relaxation is a bonus as well.

## YOU WILL NEED

- 2 tablespoons fuller's earth

- 2 teaspoons (approximately) of warm water

- 1 tablespoon lavender flowers

- 1-2 litres of hot water

- A large towel

- A place to relax with feet elevated

1. Stir water into fuller's earth until a smooth, sticky paste is formed. Add a few drops more water if necessary. Set aside.

2. Soak the lavender flowers in a pot with about a litre of cold water, and slowly bring to a simmer. Maintain heat for 5 minutes, then turn off stove.

3. Pull your hair back from your face and pin or tie a scarf around it. Follow steps 1-3 of cleansing routine (page 11).

4. Sit at your table with the infusion in front of you and the towel covering your head. Carefully arrange the towel so that it traps the steam and forms a tent. Position your face at a comfortable distance from the infusion and allow the steam to envelop it. This opens the pores and softens the skin. Continue the treatment for about 5 minutes until the infusion cools. Dry your face.

5. With your fingertips, pat the clay mixture over your face and neck. Do not apply to eye area. Once it is applied you must keep your facial muscles still - no smiling or talking.

6. Lie on the couch with your feet elevated on a couple of cushions. Read if it relaxes you, or just close your eyes and rest for at least a half-hour. The mask will keep working until it is totally dry, so don't rush it - and don't answer the doorbell!

7. Rinse off mask.

8. Follow Steps 4-6 of cleansing routine (pages 11-12).

This is deep-cleaning for the skin, and only needs to be done once a week. See page 23 for interim "quick masks".

## OTHER HERBAL STEAMS
## FOR DRY SKIN

❖ Chamomile, borage, elderflower, yarrow, calendula, comfrey.

# MASK FOR NORMAL/OILY SKIN

◆ ◆ ◆

This mask is made with a volcanic clay called zeolite. It has the unusual ability of ion transference, which means that it can pull dirt and poisons out of many substances, including skin. Ideal for teenage skin.

## YOU WILL NEED

- 2 tablespoons volcanic clay

- 2 tablespoons (approximately) warm water

- 1 tablespoon field horsetail

- About a litre of hot water

- A large towel

- A place to relax with your feet elevated

1. Stir water into clay until a smooth, sticky paste is blended. Add a few more drops of water if necessary, enough that it will stick on your skin without being too runny. Set aside.

2. Drop the horsetail into about a litre of boiling water and simmer for ten minutes. Leave covered on very low heat.

3. Pull your hair back from your face and pin or tie it securely. Cover with a scarf tied at the back.

4. Follow steps 1-3 (inclusive) of cleansing routine on page 11. Sit with the hot infusion in front of you and the towel over your head. Carefully arrange the towel so that it forms a little tent to trap the steam and direct it to your face. This will open the pores and soften the skin. Continue steam treatment for about ten minutes until mixture cools. Carefully dry your face.

5. With the tips of your fingers, pat mask over your face and neck, but avoid eye areas. Once it is applied, you must not move your face at all. No smiling or talking.

6. Lie on the couch with your feet elevated on a couple of cushions. Read if you want, or just keep your eyes closed with a couple of moist tea bags over them. Rest for at least half an hour until the mask is totally hard and dry. As it dries and shrinks, it will pull microscopic impurities from your skin. It will also create heat, which stimulates circulation. Let it dry thoroughly.

7. Rinse off mask with warm water.

8. Follow steps 4-6 inclusive of cleansing routine on pages 11-12. If you have especially oily skin, go back to step 1 and repeat the whole routine.

◆ ◆ ◆

Normal skin will not need the deep-clean treatment more than once a week. Very oily or troubled skin may benefit from more frequent treatments.

## OTHER HERBAL STEAMS FOR NORMAL/OILY SKIN

❖ Sage, horsetail, apple cider vinegar, mint, rose petals, rose hips, lemongrass, red zinger tea.

# QUICK PICK-UP MASKS

◆ ◆ ◆

If you don't have time for the full treatment, these will please your skin.

## MIX TOGETHER AND APPLY:

- ❖ A beaten egg plus 1 tablespoon of brewers' yeast

- ❖ 1 tablespoon honey plus 2 tablespoons of cooked, strained oatmeal

- ❖ 1 tablespoon yoghurt plus 1 tablespoon of pureed strawberries

- ❖ 3 tablespoons mashed papaya

- ❖ 1 tablespoon honey plus 1 tablespoon mashed avocado

- ❖ I tablespoon honey plus 2 tablespoons pureed grapes

- ❖ 3 tablespoons pureed tomato

- ❖ 1 tablespoon yoghurt plus 2 tablespoons pureed cucumber

◆ ◆ ◆

Leave on for at least 15 minutes. Wash as usual.

## Help for oily skin

❖ Brewers' yeast, apple cider vinegar, yoghurt, wheat germ, crushed almonds, salt, bran

## Help for dry skin

❖ Avocado, papaya, egg yolk, lecithin, honey, corn milk, dried apricots

## Skin softeners

❖ Cucumber, papaya, aloe vera, comfrey, grapes

*"Women are like tea bags. They don't know how strong they are until they get into hot water."*

*Eleanor Roosevelt*

# SAFE SUNSCREEN

◆ ◆ ◆

Does not contain hydroxy methoxy methyl benzophen-
one, isopropyl dibenzoylmethane, octyl dimethyl
paraminobenzoate, or any other scary things.

### INGREDIENTS

- 2 tablespoons emu oil

- 1 tablespoon sesame oil

- 3 tablespoons grapeseed oil

- 3 tablespoons soya/cottonseed oil

- 1 tablespoon coated titanium dioxide

- 6 tablespoons 4x tea

- 1 tablespoon aloe vera gel

- 3 tablespoons distilled water

1. Make 4x tea by simmering a tea bag in two cups of
   water in an open pot until the liquid is reduced to 1/2
   cup.  Allow to cool and remove tea bag.

2. Combine oils and stir over low heat until they melt
   together.  Stir in titanium dioxide.

3. In a separate pot, combine 4x tea with aloe vera gel. With both mixtures at a lukewarm temperature, add oils to liquids, stirring until blended. Beat on low until cool and creamy.

4. Add water a little at a time, beating on high until mixture is the consistency of whipped cream.

5. Put in small sterilised jars and refrigerate when not in use. Extra jars can be frozen until needed.

◆ ◆ ◆

Makes about 1 1/4 cups of velvety cream.

### WHY?

- ❖ **Emu oil** to pamper your skin.

- ❖ **Sesame oil**. A natural sunscreen.

- ❖ **Grapeseed oil**. Helps to prevent oxidation.

- ❖ **Soya oil**. Improves resiliency of skin.

- ❖ **Cottonseed oil**. Forms a moisture barrier.

- ❖ **Titanium Dioxide** is a natural pigment that blocks the sun's rays.

- ❖ **4x Tea.** Tea contains tannin, a natural sunscreen.

- ❖ **Aloe Vera Gel**. A natural sunscreen and burn preventative.

- ❖ **Distilled Water** because your skin needs it.

**N O T E S**

*Remember the Kiwi / Aussie rules for sun:*

***Slip, Slop, Slap!***

*Slip on a shirt ~ Slop on some sunscreen ~ Slap on a hat.*

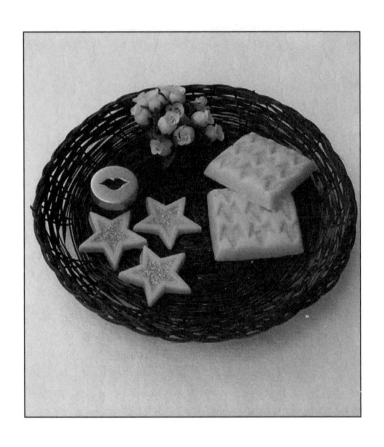

# CREAMS AND BUTTERS

❖ ❖ ❖

*Photo: Lip balm, ylang-ylang glitter bars, lavender massage bars.*

# E-MAZING EMU OIL

◆ ◆ ◆

For thousands of years the Australian Aborigines used emu oil for its healing powers. They were wise, as modern science now verifies.

Arthritis is largely absent in Aboriginal tribes, whereas about 10% of Australians currently suffer from this disease.

## EMU OIL IS:

* Anti-inflammatory, with effects comparable to ibuprofen

* Bacteriostatic (does not promote growth of bacteria)

* Hypoallergenic (not known to cause skin irritation or have any side effects)

* Highly penetrating, non-greasy

* Non-comedogenic (does not clog pores)

## Emu oil contains:

- ❖ Vitamin E, an antioxidant and healer

- ❖ Vitamin A, a known skin repairer and antioxidant

- ❖ Linoleic Acid, which eases muscle pain and joint aches

- ❖ Oleic Acid, a skin cell regenerator and anti-wrinkle agent

- ❖ Sapogens, proven skin softeners

- ❖ Terpines, known antiseptics

◆ ◆ ◆

There is a great deal of information about emu oil on the worldwide web. It has many therapeutic connotations for such conditions as arthritis, eczema and carpal tunnel syndrome, as well as for burns and scars. Beneficial as a massage oil for people and pets, too.

The oil I use comes from the Outback Emu Ranch on Vancouver Island. The birds are raised for their gourmet meat, but they also have a fat storage pad, almost like a little hump, on their backs. This is the main source of the wonderful oil. It is rendered at a special processing plant to cosmetic specifications, a complex process that is carefully monitored and regulated.

The finished oil is expensive, but does not have to be used full strength. About 20% emu oil in the fat/oil content of a formulation gives you all of its benefits.

As well as regenerating, softening and conditioning your skin, the oil prevents moisture loss by forming a protective barrier. It has no known harmful side effects, and has been tested by the Aborigines for several thousand years!

# ELEGANT EMU MOISTURISER

◆ ◆ ◆

An all-purpose, 'nose to toes' type moisturiser.  Safe for any skin!  This is the only moisturiser you will ever need.

### YOU WILL NEED

- ◆ 2 tablespoons emu oil

- ◆ 4 tablespoons soya/cottonseed oil

- ◆ 3 tablespoons grapeseed oil, macerated with calendula petals (page 48)

- ◆ 1 tablespoon honey, preferably unpasteurised

- ◆ 2 tablespoons apple, carrot, noni or pineapple juice

- ◆ 4 tablespoons lemon juice

- ◆ A few drops essential oil, if desired.

- ◆ 3 tablespoons distilled or boiled water (cold)

1. Combine oils and stir over low heat until blended.

2. In a separate pot, blend fruit juice and honey, stirring until honey melts.  Too much heat will destroy the enzymes, so keep it low.

3. Remove both pots from heat and cool until the contents are approximately the same temperature.

4. Add oils to juice mixture, stirring by hand until absorbed. Continue to stir until cool, then place in freezer for about 4 minutes until chilled.

5. Whip on 'high', adding essential oil and distilled water, a little at a time, until the mixture is the consistency of whipped cream.

6. Put into small well-washed jars (baby food jars or smaller).

7. Keep refrigerated. Extra jars can be frozen until you are ready to use them, but do not re-freeze once cream thaws.

◆ ◆ ◆

Refrigeration is necessary as no chemical preservatives are used. Makes up to 1 1/3 cups of all purpose moisturiser.

## WHY?

- ❖ **Emu oil** is the closest to human sebum. Penetrates and moisturises.

- ❖ **Soy oil** stabilises and forms a protective barrier.

- ❖ **Cottonseed oil** moisturises and preserves.

- ❖ **Grapeseed oil** is light textured with natural preservative qualities.

- ❖ **Honey** moisturises, soothes and heals.

- ❖ **Water** is the thing your skin needs most.

- ❖ **Calendula** tones and soothes.

- ❖ **Juices** gently P.H. balance your skin.

# HEALING LIP BALM

◆ ◆ ◆

A down-to-earth lip balm to solve the dry, sore, cracked, chapped lips problem once and for all.

Based on therapeutic emu oil.

### INGREDIENTS

- 1 tablespoon olive oil
- 1 tablespoon sesame oil
- 2 tablespoon grapeseed oil
- 2 tablespoons emu oil
- 1 tablespoon beeswax
- 1/4 teaspoon honey
- 2 drops tea tree essential oil (if desired)

1. Wash lip balm tubes with warm, soapy water and rinse well. Allow to dry thoroughly.

2. Set tubes into a bed of clean sand, uncooked rice or any granular substance that will support them. This will make pouring much easier.

3. Melt beeswax in a double boiler or a clean can set in a pot of water. Add other oils and stir until combined. Do not overheat.

4. Add tea tree essential oil.

5. Pour very carefully into tubes and allow to set. Leftover mixture can be stored in the fridge and re-melted when needed.

◆ ◆ ◆

Makes 3 1/2 ounces of gentle but persistent moisturiser, medicated with tea tree essential oil if desired. Fills approximately 20 tubes.

# LIP BUTTER

◆ ◆ ◆

Based on the ultimate moisturiser - emu oil, luscious lip butter solves the problem of dry lips beautifully.

## INGREDIENTS

- 2 tablespoons emu oil

- 2 tablespoons sweet almond oil

- 2 tablespoons grapeseed oil

- 2 tablespoons sesame oil

- 1 tablespoon beeswax

- 1/2 - 1 teaspoon flavour oil

- Cosmetic glitter if desired

1. Wash container pots very thoroughly in warm soapy water. If the pots are plastic, do not actually boil them, as they may shrink! Rinse well and allow to dry thoroughly.

2. Melt beeswax in a double boiler with other oils and stir until combined. Do not overheat.

3. Add flavour oil. Pour carefully into small, clean, 5 g or 10 g pots (1 or 2 teaspoons).

4. If you are using glitter, sprinkle a little on the bottom of your pots, and pour 1/2 full. Allow to set, sprinkle more glitter and fill. When firm, top with one more sprinkle of glitter and cap. This is fiddly, but the glitter will not distribute itself any other way.

◆ ◆ ◆

Makes 1/2 cup or 24 five-gram pots of luscious lip butter.

# BIG LAVENDER
# MASSAGE BARS

◆  ◆  ◆

Use for a relaxing body or foot massage.

### INGREDIENTS

- 3 tablespoons beeswax

- 2 tablespoons shea butter

- 1 tablespoon unsalted butter

- 1 tablespoon sunflower oil

- 3 tablespoons emu oil

- 2 tablespoons grapeseed oil

- 1/2 teaspoon lavender essential oil

1. Carefully melt beeswax in a double boiler or a water bath. Add other oils and stir until melted and combined. Do not overheat.

2. Remove from heat and add lavender E.O.

3. Pour into molds* (metal or plastic) and allow to set.

*Small soap, chocolate or jello molds can be used. Muffin pans, mini loaf pans or novelty pans will work. Pudding cups, partially filled, make useful molds, as do Sheba cat food containers.

◆ ◆ ◆

Makes about 6 ounces, enough for three large bars.

# YLANG-YLANG GLITTER BARS

◆ ◆ ◆

Delicate massage bars, spiced with glitter and perfumed with the evocative fragrance of ylang-ylang essential oil.

## INGREDIENTS

- 3 tablespoons beeswax

- 2 tablespoons soya/cottonseed oil

- 2 tablespoons cocoa butter

- 2 tablespoons emu oil

- 1 tablespoon olive oil

- 2 tablespoons sweet almond oil

- 1/2 teaspoon ylang-ylang essential oil

- Cosmetic glitter

1. Carefully melt beeswax and oils in a double boiler or a water bath, and stir until melted and combined. Do not overheat.

2. Remove from heat and stir in ylang-ylang.

3. Sprinkle bottoms of molds lightly with glitter. Pour 1/2 full and allow to become firm. Sprinkle with glitter again and pour top part of molds. Leave until firm and top with one more sprinkle of glitter. (If you try to put glitter in with the main mixture, it will not spread evenly).

N.B. Try to find small, dainty molds for these bars and only use about 1 tablespoon (or less) of mixture for each.

◆ ◆ ◆

Makes 3/4 cup (6 ounces), approximately 12 small bars.

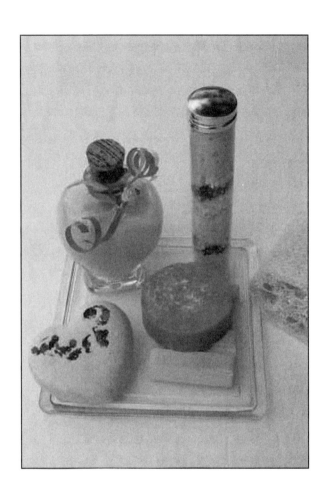

# BATH BLISS

❖  ❖  ❖

*Photo: Manna, crushed bath bombs, bath blessing, goat's milk soap, loofah.*

# MANNA BATH LOTION

◆ ◆ ◆

Not just a floating film, this lotion blends with your bath water and soaks luxuriously into your skin.

## INGREDIENTS

- ◆ 1 tablespoon oat flakes
- ◆ 1 tablespoon barley flakes
- ◆ 3 cups water
- ◆ 1/4 cup pure vegetable soap, grated
- ◆ 1 cup water
- ◆ 1 1/2 tablespoons liquid lecithin
- ◆ 2 tablespoons sunflower oil
- ◆ A few drops of your favourite essential oil

1. Simmer oats and barley in 3 cups water, covered, for 15 minutes. Stir and strain through muslin or an old nylon. Squeeze out as much of the creamy 'gel' as possible and stir into liquid. Discard remainder of flakes. Set liquid aside to cool.

2. Add grated soap to 1 cup water. Bring to a gentle boil and simmer for 5 minutes.

3. To soap solution, add sunflower oil and liquid lecithin. Simmer and stir until combined. Remove from heat.

4. When both mixtures are approximately the same temperature (cool enough to put your finger in) beat soap solution on medium for 2 minutes.

5. Slowly add 1/2 cup of oatmeal solution to the soap mixture while beating on medium speed. When mixture is smooth, reverse and pour slowly back into the rest of the oatmeal solution, continuing to beat until quite cool.

6. Add your favourite essential oil and pour into pretty bottles. Keep lotion in the fridge and shake before using.

7. Use about 1/3 cup per bath.

◆ ◆ ◆

Makes about 3 cups of sensational, soothing lotion.

**N o t e s**
*Water is the single most important thing you can put on your skin.*
*Always mist before you moisturise.*

# BATH BLESSINGS

◆ ◆ ◆

Sometimes called 'bath bombs', these are the amazing fragrant little balls that bubble and fizz about in your tub, soothing your skin and softening the water.  This basic recipe can be made in many variations.

### INGREDIENTS

- ◆ 2/3 cup baking soda

- ◆ 1/3 cup citric acid

- ◆ 1/3 cup corn starch

- ◆ 2 tablespoons grapeseed oil

- ◆ 1/2 tablespoon water

- ◆ Food colouring

- ◆ A few drops of essential oil if desired

- ◆ Flower petals or glitter to decorate

1. Combine dry ingredients and sieve together until thoroughly blended.

2. Combine wet ingredients and stir (the oil and water will not blend smoothly, but it will work out alright).

3. Drizzle wet mix over dry ingredients. Work quickly, as the liquid will cause a reaction to begin. Stir, then use your fingertips and crumble mixture together. It should be crumbly, not solid.

4. Spoon into small molds (plastic cookie cutters are fine) and pack in tightly with your fingertips. If you are using flowers to decorate, place them at the bottom of your mold and pack mixture around them.

5. Allow to dry before removing from molds. This may take a few hours, depending on thickness of molds.

6. Save any crumbs and put in a pretty bottle for extra luxurious bath salts. If you have any breakages while un-molding, crush (put in a plastic bag and crunch with a rolling pin) or crumble into a clear container. This is effective when layered with dried blossoms, sea salt, etc.

◆ ◆ ◆

Makes three very large, or eight cookie-sized, bath blessings.

**N O T E S**
*Synthetic fragrances and even most essential oils should not be used by pregnant women or on babies less than a year old.*

# BATH TEAS (INGENUI-TEAS)

◆ ◆ ◆

For those of you who don't really want to fish the rose petals out of your tub before you pull the plug, bath teas are a pretty and practical alternative. Not the ones that look like crumbled weeds in oversized tea bags, but your own creations, beauties that look as good as they smell.

## INGREDIENTS

- 1/2 cup dried rose petals
- 1/4 cup dried lavender blossoms
- 1/4 cup dried calendula petals
- 1/2 cup dried violet leaves
- 1/4 cup dried comfrey leaves
- 1/2 cup dried elderberry leaves
- Your favourite essential oil
- A nylon tulle bath scrubby*
- Ribbons and dried flowers

* Bath scrubbies are those fluffy balls that you often get given for presents along with soap. I never use them as I do not like scrubbing myself with nylon, so there were a few of them hanging on my shower hooks waiting

patiently to be noticed. Now, if you cut the cord that holds them together, you will find an amazing two metres or more of tulle tubing. Wash the dust off it and cut into approximately 12-inch lengths. Then...

1. Combine flowers and leaves carefully, without crumbling them. These herbs are only a suggestion; be creative and make your own mix from available leaves and blossoms. Sprinkle essential oil over mix and cover until ready to use.

2. Take a length of your scrubby, and, with a big-eyed darning needle, thread fine ribbon or embroidery floss through the bottom, pull tight and finish with a bow. You now have a bag.

3. Fill with about 1/3 cup herbal mixture. Tie the top, leaving a loop to hang over the tap.

4. Decorate with more ribbon and flowers.

5. Hang from your tap or toss into your tub while the water is running, and let it soak while you do. Afterwards, you may wish to empty the herbs and re-use the tulle and ribbons.

6. These ingredients are only a suggestion. Herbs and scents can be varied according to your preference. Other things you may enjoy using are: chamomile, orange peel, elderberries, rosehips, mint, borage, nasturtiums, sunflower petals... the list is up to you.

◆ ◆ ◆

Quite simple to make and so much prettier than the usual monster tea bags, which hide their dainty contents.  Recyclable too.

# FLOWER WATERS

◆ ◆ ◆

So simple to make, and a beneficial addition to your facial routine.

## YOU WILL NEED

- ◆ A spray mister bottle made of blue, green or amber glass (essential oils will eat plastic)

- ◆ Distilled water

- ◆ Essential oil of your choice

1. Choose your essential oil, being careful to do an allergy test (page 56) if you have not used it before.

2. For each tablespoon of distilled water, add 1-2 drops of essential oil.

3. Put in spray mister and shake well before each use. Use in place of plain distilled water when you do your face-wash routine.

◆ ◆ ◆

# Benefits of Some Essential Oils

- **Eczema and psoriasis:** Bergamot, geranium, patchouli.

- **Acne:** Camphor, cedarwood, clary sage, grapefruit, juniper berry, lavender, lemon, litsea cubeba, niaouli, orange, palmarosa, rose geranium, rosemary, sage, tea tree. Inflamed skin: chamomile, lavender, rose absolute, ylang ylang.

- **Dry and mature skin:** Frankincense, jasmine, myrrh, neroli, rose absolute.

- **Insect repellant:** Basil, cedarwood, citronella, clove leaf, eucalyptus, lavender, lemon, litsea cubeba, rosemary.

- **Aphrodisiac:** Ginger, patchouli, ylang ylang.

◆ ◆ ◆

If you are pregnant, essential oils are not for you. Use pure, distilled water for hydration.

Synthetically manufactured fragrances are chemical compounds designed to stimulate us. They contain a plethora of toxic ingredients and are a major cause of allergies.

Essential oils should be used with discretion after you have studied their properties. They can be very beneficial, but study their properties before you buy and use them.

# SEA SALT SEAWEED SCRUB

◆ ◆ ◆

For the mermaid in all of us... a refreshing, slightly slippery scrub.

### INGREDIENTS

- 1/2 cup sunflower oil
- 1 tablespoon liquid lecithin
- 2/3 cup coarse sea salt
- 1 teaspoon dulse, chopped fine
- 1 teaspoon kelp powder
- 1/4 teaspoon spirulina

1. Melt oil, lecithin and spirulina over low heat and whisk with a fork until thoroughly blended.

2. Mix in kelp powder and dulse.

3. Pour over salt and combine well.

4. Store in small glass jars (1/2 cup) in fridge.

◆ ◆ ◆

## To use

❖ Take a hot shower. Turn off the water but stay in the tub and massage the mixture briskly, a bit at a time, over every bit of bare skin. Turn the water back on and rinse without soap. Now (yikes!) a cold splash and towel dry.

◆ ◆ ◆

A pick-me-up for your skin and your psyche.

# EVE'S EDIBLE OIL

◆ ◆ ◆

Eden was never so delectable. A tempting massage oil, apple flavoured.

## INGREDIENTS

- ◆ 6 tablespoons grapeseed oil

- ◆ 2 tablespoons sweet almond oil

- ◆ 4 tablespoons sunflower oil

- ◆ 2 teaspoons Sweet Apple flavour oil*

*For something different, try any of the lip balm edible flavourings. You will find everything from pina colada to chocolate mint, as well as lots of fruit flavours.

1. Measure all ingredients into a pretty bottle.

2. Do not heat. Just cap and shake well.

3. Store in the fridge.

---

**ALLERGY TESTING**
*To test for allergies, simply put a little of the ingredient on the inner part of your elbow and cover with a band-aid. Leave overnight. If there is any redness or irritation, don't use the ingredient.*

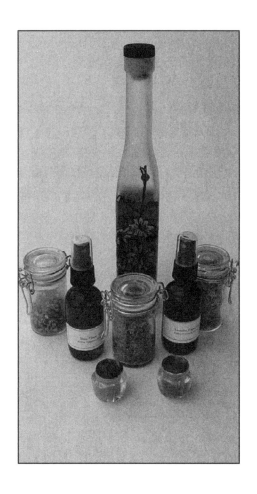

# HERBAL HELPERS

*Photo: Alcanet root extract, elderberries, lavender water, lavender blossoms, rose water, calendula petals. cream perfumes.*

# ESSENTIAL OILS

◆ ◆ ◆

Aromatherapy is a complex subject, full of variables. The rule of thumb is, "if you like an essential oil, it is probably good for you". But before making decisions on therapeutic uses of oils, read everything you can find and, most important, talk to a qualified aromatherapist. "Qualified" means certificated by an appropriate organisation. Aromatherapy is a serious science, not a whim, so ask the experts.

Be careful to read the labels when buying essential oils. Many of them are diluted by 10% or more in carrier oils, and small print is **very** small on a tiny 10 ml bottle. Essential oils vary enormously from product to product, brand to brand, or even (like wine) from year to year.

My aromatherapist tells me that there are only three people in the world, at this time, who are qualified to select, judge and grade essential oils. Because of variations in weather and soil, what was best in France last year may be great in Turkey in the current season. We don't know this when we pick up a bottle, so it pays to do some research. These oils need birth certificates!

It is not always possible to make essential oil from different types of plants and some things are sold as essential oils that are actually extracts.

Vanilla is one of these - it smells wonderful, but it is not an essential oil, and you may have difficulty blending it with oil-based recipes.

Fragrances are divided into three categories.

❖ *Base or bottom notes* - evaporate slowly, have a soothing effect and are generally extracted from gums or woods.

❖ *Middle notes* - aid digestion and metabolism and come from spices and some herbs.

❖ *Top notes* - are stimulating and uplifting, but quite volatile. They include citrus, sage and eucalyptus

◆ ◆ ◆

The following list of essential oils is not comprehensive, but does give some idea of the varied effects of E.O. I have included an approximate cost for average quality of each type, but you will probably pay far more for premium quality.

| Essential Oil | Properties | CDN $/10 ml (approximate) |
|---|---|---|
| *Bergamot* | May help eczema and psoriasis. Good for stress. Top note | $11.95 |

| Essential Oil | Properties | CDN $/10 ml (approximate) |
|---|---|---|
| *Chamomile (Moroccan)* | Helpful for dermatitis and inflamed skin. Middle note. | $29.95 |
| *Clary Sage* | Aids acne, oily skin or hair, wrinkles. Antiseptic, sedative  Top/middle note. | $11.50 |
| *Fennel* | For bruises, mature skin, cellulite. Stimulates circulation. | $10.50 |
| *Frankincense* | For dry and mature skin, scars, blemishes. Bottom note. | $26.95 |
| *Jasmine Absolute* | Especially good for dry, sensitive skin. Bottom note. | $105.50 |
| *Lavender* | For allergies, dermatitis, burns, insect bites, deodorant. Top/middle note. | $10.50 |
| *Lemon* | For brittle nails, oily skin, varicose veins, warts, arthritis. A natural deodorant. Top note. | $8.95 |
| *Litsea Cubeba* | For dermatitis, oily skin. An insect repellent. Top note. | $7.95 |

| Essential Oil | Properties | CDN $/10 ml (approximate) |
|---|---|---|
| Melissa | For allergies, insect bites and insect repellent. Top note. | $145.50 |
| Myrrh | For mature complexions and chapped or dry skin. Bottom note. | $28.79 |
| Neroli | For poor circulation, stretch marks, dry skin. Bottom note. | $109.50 |
| Orange | Antiseptic, good for oily skin and for stress. Top note. | $6.59 |
| Patchouli | Good for chapped skin, wrinkles, eczema. Natural deodorant. Bottom note. | $17.25 |
| Peppermint | Antiseptic and stimulant. Good for acne. Top note. | $7.25 |
| Rose Geranium | Use for dull, oily skin. Stimulates circulation. Top/middle note. | $15.90 |
| Rose Absolute | For allergies, bruises and dry, mature skin. Bottom note. | $134.05 |

| Essential Oil | Properties | CDN $/10 ml (approximate) |
|---|---|---|
| *Tea Tree* | Antibacterial, antiseptic and deodorant. | $10.50 |
| *Ylang Ylang* | For oily or irritated skin. An anti-depressant. Middle/bottom note. | $14.95 |

# HERBAL PREPARATIONS

◆ ◆ ◆

## MACERATION

❖ Herbs are added to oil, vinegar or wine, and kept in a
cool, dark place for two to four weeks. Mixture
should be shaken every few days, and strained when
ready. The liquid is used and the herbs discarded.
Dried plant material is more effective than fresh in a
maceration.

## DECOCTION

❖ Put fresh or dried herbs in a pot of cold water, using
about a tablespoon of herbs per cup of water. Cover
and bring to boil slowly, then simmer for fifteen
minutes. Allow to stand, covered, for a further ten
minutes before straining. A decoction is meant to be
used soon after it is made.

## INFUSION

❖ Tea is an infusion, but it can be made with many
herbs, either fresh or dried. Place the herbs in a
heavy ceramic teapot that has been previously
warmed. Add boiling water, and cover for about ten
minutes before pouring.

# ENFLEURAGE

❖ In past centuries, flower petals were soaked in hot fat, and steeped for several days, with more and more petals added until the fat was saturated.

❖ When the fat cooled, it solidified and the essential oil from the petals formed a separate layer. This was washed with alcohol, and yielded an 'absolute' - a thick, concentrated oil.

# CREAM PERFUME

◆ ◆ ◆

If you crave the luxury of essential oils, here is the best way to make your very own personal fragrance.

## INGREDIENTS

- ◆ 1 tablespoon grapeseed oil

- ◆ 1 tablespoon cocoa butter

- ◆ 1/2 teaspoon beeswax

- ◆ 1/8 teaspoon pink clay

- ◆ 1 teaspoon (approximately) essential oil

1. Heat oil and beeswax in a small metal container set into a pot of hot water (an ordinary double boiler is too big for this amount, so you need to improvise). Keep heat low enough to prevent water from boiling up into the oils. Stir frequently.

2. When beeswax is melted, add pink clay and blend well.

3. Add your choice of essential oils. You may decide to use a single fragrance or a blend. Whichever you choose, it is wise to do an allergy test first (see page 56).

4. Spoon into small, decorative pots (sterilised with boiling water) and cap firmly. Extra pots may be kept in the fridge, but do not need to be frozen. Grapeseed oil contains a natural preservative and keeps well as long as it is cool.

5. Smooth perfume cream onto your pulse points and use often.

Good essential oil is therapeutic and can either relax or invigorate you. Make some for every mood!

### Why?

- ❖ **Grapeseed oil:** A fine base oil containing a natural preservative.

- ❖ **Cocoa butter:** Holds fragrance well. May clog pores if used as a face cream, but is good for body and pulse points.

- ❖ **Beeswax:** Crystaline structure binds cream to a firm consistency.

- ❖ **Pink Clay:** Used for colour. Non-invasive and harmless to your skin.

- ❖ **Essential Oil:** See pages 59-61.

# CALENDULA / GRAPESEED MACERATION

◆ ◆ ◆

May be used as it is as a gentle healing oil, or can be incorporated into more complex recipes.

### INGREDIENTS

- 4 ounces grapeseed oil at room temperature
- 2 tablespoons dried calendula petals

1. Place both ingredients in a jar, cover and put in a cool, dark cupboard for three weeks.  Shake or stir every few days.

2. When ready, strain petals, squeezing out as much oil as possible.  Discard petals and keep oil refrigerated until you are ready to use it.

3. This method is equally effective for dried elderberry blossoms, violets, rose petals, and a variety of herbs.

◆ ◆ ◆

Works best with dried plant material.

# ELDERFLOWER CREAM

◆ ◆ ◆

Elderberry bushes grow wild throughout much of southern Canada and the U.S. Flowers, berries and leaves all have useful cosmetic properties.

### INGREDIENTS

- A big bowl of fresh elderflowers

- About a pound (1/2 kg.) of vegetable shortening

- 2 tablespoons honey

1. Strip elderflowers from their stems.

2. Melt the shortening in a heavy pot and add as many flowers as it can cover.

3. Do not boil, but keep on a low simmer for an hour. Strain out flowers and use for compost.

4. Add honey to the hot oil and stir until it is thoroughly melted and combined.

5. Pour into well-washed pots and keep in a cool place.

◆ ◆ ◆

This is a soothing, healing cream for baby rashes. Moms will enjoy it as well.

# CALENDULA CREAM

◆　◆　◆

Use the English marigolds rather than the South African variety.  Their properties are more beneficial to your skin.

### YOU WILL NEED

- A 1 litre measuring cup filled with calendula flowers

- Approximately 1 litre of hot water

- 1 pound (1/2 kg.) vegetable shortening

- Small sterilised glass pots or tins.

1. Place flowers in hot water and simmer for 2 hours with lid on pot.

2. Add shortening and continue to cook very gently uncovered.

3. When all the water has evaporated strain off the flowers and pot the cream.

◆　◆　◆

An effective ointment for burns, and a generally good antiseptic.

# DANDRUFF RINSE

◆ ◆ ◆

Combines the bacterial-fighting qualities of sage and birch with antiseptic tea tree oil. Rosemary stimulates and regenerates skin and hair.

## YOU WILL NEED

- ◆ 1/2 cup dried sage

- ◆ 1 litre of water.

- ◆ A few drops rosemary essential oil

- ◆ A few drops tea tree essential oil

- ◆ A few drops birch essential oil (optional)

1. Harvest sage leaves and blossoms when plant is in full bloom. Dry indoors on flat trays. When completely dry, store in jars in a cool place.

2. Take 1/2 cup sage and make a decoction by simmering in water for 20 minutes, allowing to steep for a further hour, then straining away the plant material.

3. Add essential oils and shake well to combine.

4.  Put in a spray bottle and spray onto scalp daily for a week.  This can be done after washing hair or between washes onto dry hair.

5.  Keep decoction in the fridge between uses, and make a new one after about a week.

◆ ◆ ◆

A safer alternative to commercial dandruff shampoos.

# RINSE FOR BLONDE HAIR

◆ ◆ ◆

Chamomile and horsetail soften, calendula and clover add highlights, lemon juice or vinegar adjust PH balance and nettle stimulates hair growth.

### You will need

- ◆ 2 tablespoons chamomile

- ◆ 2 tablespoons calendula flowers

- ◆ 2 tablespoons red clover blossoms

- ◆ 2 tablespoons field horsetail

- ◆ 2 tablespoons nettle (optional)

- ◆ 1 litre distilled water

- ◆ 1/4 cup of lemon juice or apple cider vinegar

1. These quantities are for freshly picked herbs. If you use dried ones, reduce their amounts by one third.

2. Place horsetail in water and simmer, covered, for about a half hour.

3. Add the rest of the herbs and continue to simmer gently for a further 20 minutes.

4. Steep for an hour with lid on pot.  Strain off herbs and use in compost.

5. Add lemon juice or vinegar and pour into clean jar or bottle.

6. Keep in fridge and shake before using.  If you wish to make larger quantities, freeze the extra containers.

❖ ❖ ❖

Apply to hair as a final rinse. Do not wash out.

# RINSE FOR DARK HAIR

◆ ◆ ◆

Purifies hair and skin.  Horsetail softens and smooths, while walnut shells highlight hair without damaging it.

## INGREDIENTS

- 2 tablespoons sage
- 2 tablespoons rosemary
- 2 tablespoons field horsetail
- 2 tablespoons walnut shells
- 2 tablespoons birch leaves (optional)
- 2 bay leaves
- 2 litres distilled water

1. This recipe uses fresh herbs.  If you have dried ones, reduce their quantities by one-third.

2. Place walnut shells, horsetail and rosemary in a heavy pot with water.  Simmer, covered, for an hour.

3. Add sage, burdock and bay leaves, and simmer for a further 20 minutes.

4. Allow to steep, covered, for another hour.

5. Strain off plant material and bottle in sterilised containers. Keep in the fridge. Extra containers can be frozen.

◆ ◆ ◆

Apply to hair as a final rinse. Do not wash out.

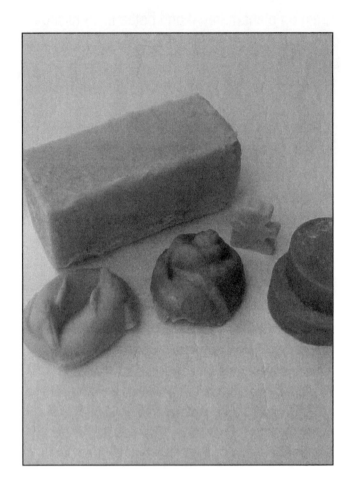

# HOMEMADE SOAP

*Photo: Rough-cut soap block, molded soap, floating flower soap, teddy-bear cut soap, goat's milk soap.*

# SOAP FROM SCRATCH

◆  ◆  ◆

A simple basic recipe that can be customised to your own choice.

### EQUIPMENT

- ❖ A large pot, stainless steel or enamel
- ❖ A strong, plastic, 2-litre jug
- ❖ A candy thermometer
- ❖ A stick blender
- ❖ Rubber gloves and glasses or goggles
- ❖ Old newspaper
- ❖ A plastic or wooden spoon
- ❖ 3 or 4 clean 1-litre milk cartons or round potato chip containers.

### INGREDIENTS

- ◆ 1 3 lb can of vegetable shortening
- ◆ 1 litre distilled water
- ◆ 28.5 ounces of olive oil (Pomace grade)
- ◆ 1 can (9.5 ounces) Gillette's Lye

1. Measure and melt together the 3 lb can of vegetable shortening and the same can half full of olive oil. Heat to approximately 110 degrees F.

2. At the same time add your can of lye (9.5 ounces) to 1 litre of distilled water. Wear gloves for this, and don't breathe the stuff. Only do this in a well-ventilated room. Stir with wooden spoon and let the mixture cool until it is approximately the same temperature as the oil.

3. Add lye mix to oil mix while stirring with wooden spoon (use gloves). Use stick blender on high until soap traces, or forms a visible trail when you stir it. Rest blender every couple of minutes and stir by hand. Those things are not built to go non-stop.

4. Pour into milk cartons, potato chip cartons or your choice of molds. Let rest under a blanket for at least 48 hours.

5. Cut into bars and allow to season (at least 4 weeks in a cool cupboard), or hand-mill it.

This recipe will fill 3 1-litre milk cartons, approximately 5 lbs of finished soap.

**N O T E S**
*Most glycerine we see on the drug store shelves is a petroleum derivative. Natural glycerine is a by-product of the soap-making process.*

# HAND-MILLING

◆ ◆ ◆

Hand-milled or French-milled soap eliminates the need for a long curing period.

### INGREDIENTS

- 6 cups of pure vegetable soap, grated

- 6 tablespoons water

- 6 tablespoons of optional ingredients if desired (herbs, spices, colour, essential oil, seeds, etc.)

1. Put grated soap and water into your slow cooker on low for about 4 hours until it looks like melted honey.

2. Add your choice of optional ingredients and combine thoroughly. Pour into molds. It will be fairly thick and more inclined to hold air bubbles, so press it down well. This soap is now 'cooked' and will be ready to use in a couple of days.

If you find the soap unwilling to leave the mold, put it in the freezer overnight. It should pop right out.

◆ ◆ ◆

❖ Possible additives for soap are: oatmeal, poppy seeds, ground lemon or orange peel, freshly ground coffee, honey, vanilla beans, various spices, essential oils.

❖ To colour your soap, try alkanet root for pink/purple, spirulina for green, tumeric or annato seeds for yellow, or cinnamon for a rich brown. Food colouring will work if you add it with water, but it fades quite fast.

❖ I do not add fragrance to any of my soaps for three reasons. First because it causes allergies in so many people, second because the choice of fragrance is highly personal (so you don't want to make a whole batch of lavender and then find that people actually want vanilla) and third because it takes a lot of expensive essential oil to perfume a batch (perfumed soap may smell gorgeous but not much of the perfume actually adheres to your skin if you wash properly!). I feel that I get better mileage and better therapy out of my essential oils by using them for bath bombs or bath oils.

Soap just naturally tries to clean everything it touches, including colours and perfumes. I find it easier to add those special touches after the process, instead of during it. Star anise, cloves, orange peel and flower petals all make wonderfully fragrant decorations. Because they are not as potent as essential oils, they are safe for babies as well. Baby soap decorated with powdered rose petals or with lavender blossoms makes a lovely gift for a small person.

# GENTLE GOAT'S MILK SOAP

❖ ❖ ❖

This is the queen of soaps, as pure and kind as an angel's kiss.

## EQUIPMENT

- ❖ A large pot, stainless steel or enamel
- ❖ A strong, plastic or glass 2 litre jug
- ❖ A candy thermometer
- ❖ A stick blender
- ❖ Rubber gloves and glasses or goggles
- ❖ Old newspaper
- ❖ A plastic or wooden spoon
- ❖ 3 or 4 clean 1 litre cartons or round potato chip containers

## INGREDIENTS

- ◆ 1 3lb can of vegetable shortening
- ◆ 28.5 ounces of olive oil (Pomace grade)
- ◆ 1 litre of goat's milk

- ◆  1 can (9.5 ounces) Gillette's lye

1. Measure and melt together the 3 lb can of vegetable shortening and the same can 1/2 full of olive oil. Heat to approximately 110 degrees F.

2. At the same time, add your can of lye very carefully to the goat's milk. Wear gloves and don't let the liquid splash up. Do this in a well-ventilated area and don't breathe the fumes.

3. Stir gently with a wooden spoon. The milk will turn bright yellow and curdled (it will look like something you should throw out, but don't panic!).

4. Let cool to same temperature as the oils, stirring from time to time.

5. Add lye mix to oil mix, while stirring with wooden or plastic spoon. The curdled milk will be inclined to splash, so hold your spout as close to the oil as possible, and be sure that your hands and clothes are protected.

6. Use a stick blender on high to combine the mixture, until soap 'traces' or forms a visible trail when stirred. Rest blender every couple of minutes and stir by hand. Tracing may happen quite fast or may take up to 10 minutes. Soap has a mind of it's own!

7. Pour into clean milk cartons, potato chip containers or your choice of molds. Snuggle warm soap under a blanket for at least 48 hours until it solidifies.

8. Cut into bars, put on clean cardboard or mesh and allow to season for at least 4 weeks. This recipe does not hand-mill well, so it needs to cure naturally for best results.

❖ ❖ ❖

Recipe will fill approximately 3 milk cartons or containers, about 5 pounds of finished soap.

# FLOATING FLOWER SOAP

❖  ❖  ❖

This soap will float because it has extra air beaten into it before it sets.  Fun for the small set.

### You will need

- ❖ 10 ounces of pure vegetable soap (Soap from Scratch, page 77)

- ❖ 1/2 cup distilled water

- ❖ A kitchen grater

- ❖ A stick blender

- ❖ Electric crock pot

- ❖ Wooden spoon

- ❖ Spatula

- ❖ Soap molds in flower shapes

1. Essential oil or colour as desired

2. Grate the soap and put in pot with water.

3. Turn crock-pot to lowest setting and leave for three to four hours, until soap has melted to the consistency of liquid honey.

4. Add colour and fragrance if desired.

5. Beat at high speed for a few minutes until the mixture thickens to a whipped consistency. Let your stick blender rest every minute or so.

6. Pour or spoon into molds and place in the freezer overnight.

7. Unmold and set on a piece of cardboard or thick plastic mesh for a few days until completely dry.

Since you have 'hand-milled' this soap it is now ready to use as soon as it is dry.

◆ ◆ ◆

**N O T E S**
*Detergent based shampoos leave your hair squeaky-clean. They also strip it of natural protection and upset the acid balance. Try to think of that squeak as the sound of your hair screaming for help!*

*Double Recipe Make 3 small*
*Tupperware @ 5 lbs each (slightly*
*less*

# SHAMPOO BARS

◆ ◆ ◆

A rich foamy bar that actually strengthens your hair.

### INGREDIENTS

- 24 ounces olive oil

- 22 ounces castor oil

- 23 ounces coconut oil

- 1 ounce jojoba oil

- 9.5 ounces lye

- 32 ounces water

- 4 teaspoons frankincense powder

- 2 ounces warm olive oil

1. Heat oils in a stainless steel or enamel pot, stirring
   until blended. Cool to approximately 115 degrees C.

*½ Recipe*

*13 oz olive oil*
*11 oz castor oil*
*11.5 oz coconut oil*
*1 ounce jojoba*

*5 oz lye*
*16 oz water*

*½ ounce*
*ess. oil*

2. Lye is very caustic. Using rubber gloves and goggles, carefully pour lye into water in a plastic jug. Stir with a plastic spoon until lye is dissolved. Set in a place where the fumes will not bother people or pets (try the bathroom with the fan on) and leave for about ten minutes. The mixture will become quite hot. Set in cold water until it is the same temperature as the oils.

3. Mix powder into oil and set aside. Make sure that oil mix and lye mix are at approximately the same temperature (110-115 C).

4. Using rubber gloves, carefully pour lye mixture into oil mixture and stir together. Take your stick blender and mix on high until soap begins to 'trace' or form a visible path as blender moves.

5. Blend in frankincense powder dissolved in warm olive oil and continue to use blender until soap is the consistency of light custard.

6. Pour into clean molds (1 litre milk cartons, round potato chip containers, etc.)

7. Wrap in a blanket and leave in a warm place for at least 48 hours until soap is set. Leave for one more day before removing from molds. Molds can be cut or torn off carefully. Wear rubber gloves as your soap can 'bite' until it is cured (two to six weeks).

8. Cut into bars and place on clean cardboard or plastic (not newspaper) in a fairly cool cupboard.

◆ ◆ ◆

Don't believe everything the ads tell you - people actually did have clean, shiny hair before chemical shampoos came on the market (look at some old photos of your grandparents). They used to brush their hair a lot more, something we have been discouraged from doing for the last four decades because "it might split your hair" (it will too, after your hair has been traumatized by chemicals for a few years). Because this bar contains castor oil, it will strengthen your hair so that you can actually brush it. Use a natural bristle brush and try 100 strokes. Great for your scalp and very therapeutic.

# SOAPSICLES

◆ ◆ ◆

Soap you can really get a grip on. It floats too!

### INGREDIENTS

- ◆ 6 cups grated vegetable soap (Page 54)

- ◆ Additives of your choice (Page 56)

### YOU WILL NEED

- ❖ 4 dowels or large craft sticks approximately 7" long

- ❖ Cardboard tube from paper towel roll

- ❖ Wax paper or freezer paper

- ❖ Duct tape

1. Follow instructions for hand-milled soap on Page 79.

2. Cut cardboard tube into 4" lengths.  Cut paper into 4" x 6" strips and roll each strip into an inner tube for the cardboard.  Tape in place.

3. Cut a paper circle for the bottom of the tube and cover with duct tape so that it is secure.

4. Place dowel or craft stick in center of roll and fill with melted soap.  Pack down well to avoid air pockets.

5. Allow to cool and put in freezer overnight.

6. Peel off cardboard, etc. and trim any rough edges.

7. If you want to make a hang-up soapsicle, drill a hole in the end of the stick and thread with cord.

# NATURAL SHAMPOO

◆ ◆ ◆

## INGREDIENTS

* 2 tablespoons soapwort root

* 1 tablespoon dried sage

* 1 tablespoon fresh nettles (optional)

* 1 1/4 cups distilled water

* 1/2 tablespoon castor oil

* 1 tablespoon aloe vera gel

* Pinch sea salt

* 1/2 teaspoon benzoin powder (optional)

1. Place herbs and water in a heavy pot and simmer, covered for 30 minutes.

2. Remove from heat and steep for another hour. Strain off plant material.

3. Put all ingredients in a blender or a large shaker bottle. Blend or shake until thoroughly combined.

4. Pour into sterilised bottles and keep cool.

5. To use, rub in well with fingertips, and leave on until you have finished your bath or shower, the longer the better.

6. Rinse thoroughly. No conditioner is necessary.

◆ ◆ ◆

This is a low-sudsing shampoo and will not make your hair 'squeaky', but it cleans gently and safely. The mixture will separate when left to stand, so shake well before using. If you wish to make a larger quantity, freeze the extra.

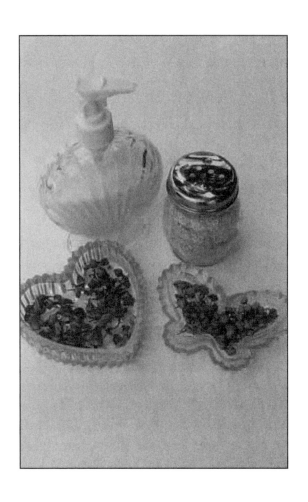

# TOP TO TOE

❖ ❖ ❖

*Photo: Liquid soap, baby powder, rose buds, tansy flowers.*

# FOOT FANTASY

◆ ◆ ◆

Cheerful feet mean a cheerful person. Try this on grumpy husbands.

### FOOT PACK

- ◆ 2 tablespoons volcanic clay

- ◆ 2 teaspoons (approximately) water

1. Make into a paste (about the consistency of liquid honey) and apply a thin layer to soles of feet and toes.

2. Elevate feet and allow pack to harden for 15-30 minutes.

3. Fill a large, flat container with warm water, and soak feet for a further 5 minutes. Use a soft scrubbing brush to remove traces of the pack. Rub feet briskly with a towel.

4. Apply Lavender Massage Bar to soles of feet and toes. Rub in firmly, paying particular attention to balls of feet, the area along the inside of each foot, and the bottoms of the toes.

## W H Y ?

❖ Your feet contain multiple nerve endings that affect every part of your body. Keep them happy!

❖ **Volcanic clay,** with its unique properties of ion exchange, draws toxins from the skin and 'sweetens' areas of application. A little volcanic clay sprinkled in shoes helps to keep them odour-free as well.

❖ **Lavender Massage Bar** soothes and softens your feet.

Save the water and leftover clay from your footbath and use it to water your plants. They will thrive on it.

◆ ◆ ◆

**N O T E S**
*It is a relief to find an ingredient that actually removes toxins from the skin. Zeolite does this very effectively. (It is also used extensively to purify commercial water systems.) It has the ability to absorb and remove loose ions.*

# FRESH MOUTHWASH

◆ ◆ ◆

An unusual flavour, but very effective.

### INGREDIENTS

- 1 tablespoon fennel seeds
- 1 tablespoon sage
- 1/4 teaspoon baking soda
- 2 teaspoons lemon juice
- 1 1/2 cups distilled water
- Food colouring if desired

1. Simmer fennel seeds in water for about 10 minutes. Turn off heat, add sage, cover and steep for a further 1/2 hour. Strain out herbs and add to your compost.

2. Take remaining liquid and stir in lemon juice and baking soda.

3. Add food colouring carefully, a drop at a time, until you are satisfied with the colour.

◆ ◆ ◆

Keep in the fridge.

# TOOTH POWDER

◆ ◆ ◆

Each of these dry ingredients has it's own cleansing abilities.  Mint adds a fresh touch.

- ◆ 1 teaspoon powdered zeolite

- ◆ 1/2 teaspoon powdered sage

- ◆ 1 teaspoon myrrh

- ◆ 1/4 teaspoon baking soda

- ◆ 6 drops mint essential oil

1. Shake or sieve dry ingredients together until thoroughly mixed.

2. Add essential oil.

3. Keep in a small, flat clean container.

4. Dip wet toothbrush into mixture and brush as usual.

**N**OTES
*Toothpaste can contain toxic ingredients. The directions on one well-known brand state that if your child swallows an amount larger than a pea, you should call the Poison Control hotline. Read the ingredient list on your toothpaste tube.*

# BABY POWDER

◆ ◆ ◆

No petroleum derivatives in this formula. Completely safe for the most precious member of the family.

## INGREDIENTS

- ◆ 1/2 cup rice flour
- ◆ 1/2 cup cornstarch
- ◆ 1/2 teaspoon emu oil or grapeseed oil
- ◆ 1 teaspoon powdered rose petals

1. To make powdered rose petals, put 1/2 cup dried petals in the blender and pulverise as finely as possible. Pour through a fine sieve to remove larger particles (these can be used in soap, bath bombs, potpourri, etc.) and separate fine powder.

2. Sift or shake together rice flour and cornstarch. Add oil, a drop at a time.

3. Put in blender with rose petal powder and process for a few seconds.

4. Pour or spoon into a pretty shaker bottle. This is a safe alternative to talc, the main ingredient of most commercial baby powder.

◆ ◆ ◆

Do not use essential oils or perfumes on babies until
they are at least a year old.

# FACE PAINT

◆ ◆ ◆

A safe and simple alternative to expensive commercial face painting sets.

## INGREDIENTS

- 1 teaspoon yoghurt
- 1 teaspoon cornstarch
- A few drops food colouring
- Glitter if desired

1. Mix yoghurt and cornstarch to a smooth paste.

2. Add food colouring a tiny bit at a time until desired colour is achieved.

3. Stir in glitter if you wish.

4. Paint a pretty little face.

◆ ◆ ◆

This face paint doubles quite efficiently as a sun block, so is a fun project for hot summer days.

# SOLID DEODORANT

◆ ◆ ◆

This is not an anti-perspirant. It works by neutralizing the bacteria that cause odour.

## INGREDIENTS

- 1 ounce beeswax

- 2 tablespoons grapeseed oil

- 1 teaspoon baking soda

- 2 tablespoons cocoa butter

- 5 drops lemon essential oil

- 5 drops patchouli essential oil

- 3 drops tea tree essential oil

- 5 drops lavender essential oil

1. Melt together oils and beeswax.

2. Stir in baking soda. Combine well.

3. Add the essential oils (if you do not like all of these varieties, or if you are allergic to them, just leave them out).

4. Pour into a clean deodorant tube (recycled is good) and allow to set.

◆ ◆ ◆

The suggested essential oils are all natural deodorants. You should test them first to make sure they agree with your system (see page 56 for allergy testing). Not for use by pregnant women or babies under one year of age.

# LIQUID HAND SOAP

◆ ◆ ◆

- ◆ 2 1/2 cups water

- ◆ 1/2 cup pure vegetable soap, grated

- ◆ 2 tablespoons corn starch

- ◆ 1/2 teaspoon gelatin, dissolved in 1/4 cup boiling water

- ◆ Essential oil if desired

1. Add grated soap to 2 cups of the cold water and bring to boil, stirring occasionally.

2. Combine the rest of the water with the cornstarch.

3. When soap is melted, stir in cornstarch mixture and dissolved gelatin. Stir thoroughly.

4. Allow to cool and pour into blender. Run on high setting for a few seconds.

5. Add any desired essential oil.

6. Pour into squeeze bottles and store extra bottles in a cool place. Shake before using.

Costs just pennies to make and is a fine replacement for detergent-based commercial hand liquids.

# PET PROTECTOR
# (FLEE FLEA!)

◆ ◆ ◆

Wash your cats, dogs and horses with shampoo made from the recipe on page 86. It will treat their hair as well and safely as it does yours.

## INGREDIENTS

- ◆ 1 cup dried tansy flowers
- ◆ 1/4 cup corn starch
- ◆ 1/2 teaspoon essential oil
- ◆ 1 teaspoon olive oil

1. Grind tansy flowers in blender until they are reduced to small particles. Put through fine sieve to separate any larger pieces.

2. Add corn starch and blend or shake well.

3. Choose any combination of the following essential oils and add to olive oil:

   - ◆ Basil, lemon, clove leaf, eucalyptus, lavender, litsea cubeba, rosemary, cedarwood, citronella

### For dogs

❖ Sprinkle powder into coat and brush in well. Sprinkle liberally on clean bedding.

### For cats

❖ Do not put onto your kitty's coat, but use lots on his or her clean bedding.

### For horses

❖ Fleas are not generally a problem, but flies are, so I call this recipe...

# FLEE FLY

◆ ◆ ◆

❖ To a cup of olive oil (the cheap pomace grade) add 1 teaspoon of your choice of the essential oils above. Try to include eucalyptus and citronella, as they are powerful mosquito repellents.

❖ Use as a wipe on entire coat, paying particular attention to insides of ears, around genitals and those places where the hair parts and the flies nibble. Be careful not to get in eyes.

◆ ◆ ◆

Olive oil is a bonus for their coats and the beastly bugs are offended by these essential oils.

**N O T E S**
*If you are using these essential oils to make insect repellent for your own personal use, be aware that some of the essential oils will act as sun sensitisers. Most of the citrus oils (lemon, litsea cubeba, citronella) can have this effect, so use with care.*

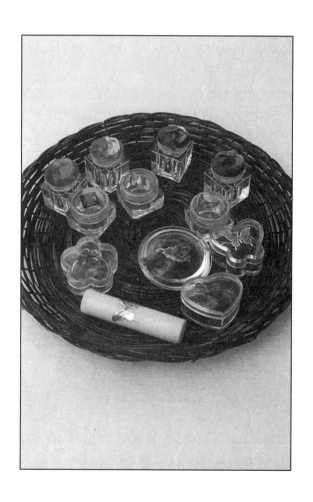

# CONTAINERS

❖  ❖  ❖

*Photo: Containers for lip balm, creams and cream perfumes.*

# CONTAINERS

◆ ◆ ◆

Good little containers for your creams, lotions and lip butters are hard to find.  Cherish your favourites, and use them over and over.

## FOR SOLIDS

By "solids" I mean anything that sets or gels, not necessarily like a rock.  I count lip butters and moisture creams as solids.  They will not react with plastic.

❖ **Glass** is easy to clean and care for, but it is expensive and cannot be safely frozen.  I try to keep one or two little glass pots on hand, but I mainly use plastic for small cosmetic items.

❖ **Plastic** comes in a variety of shapes.  Choose small containers with as smooth a finish as possible.  Wash carefully between uses.  Scrub with lots of soap, but do not boil or use very hot water.  Rinse well and dry before using.  Do not put in your dishwasher as the heat may warp them.  If the surface seems to be roughening after a few uses, discard or use for earrings or beads, etc.

◆ ◆ ◆

❖ **Glass** is attractive and safe for the things you do not wish to freeze. Look for the type of small juice bottles that have shrink-wrapped labels rather than paper or painted ones. The wrap is easily removed and the lids can be painted or decorated. Essential oils, even if they are diluted, should be kept in tinted glass to prevent deterioration.

❖ **Plastic** must be checked carefully. Some liquid products, including water, are packaged in plastic that may leach chemicals into the product. Especially insidious are 'estrogen mimics'. Tests conducted in Scandinavia have shown these to contribute to low sperm count in men and breast cancer in women. This problem is easy to avoid, as long as you know about it! Look at the bottom of the bottle. If it says HDPE or PETE it is a safe plastic for liquids. Most of the large producers of water, juice and pop are aware of this factor and package correctly, but you should always check. As far as I know, oils do not have the same leaching effect as water, but just to be sure, I always put my liquid oils and my lotions into HDPE bottles or glass.

◆ ◆ ◆

Reuse your favourite containers, pots, tubes and bottles, but be fastidious about washing and rinsing them.

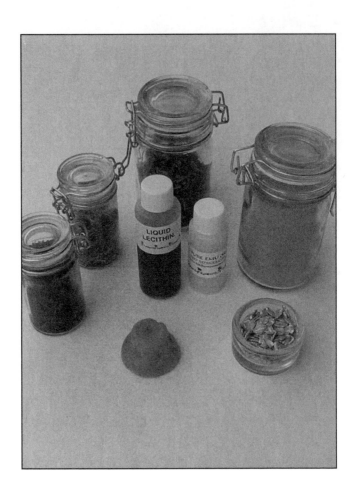

# INGREDIENTS

*Photo: lavender, calendula, sage, volcanic clay, liquid lecithin, emu oil, beeswax, oat flakes.*

# INGREDIENTS USED

◆ ◆ ◆

| Ingredient | Properties |
|---|---|
| Aloe Vera Gel | A healing anti-irritant gel. |
| Apple Cider Vinegar | Use with water as an acid rinse to adjust the P.H. of skin or hair. |
| Baking Soda | Soothing in water, slightly antiseptic, removes odours. |
| Barley Flakes | Boil and strain to make a creamy skin-soother. |
| Benzoin Powder | A natural antiseptic and preservative derived from the resin of styrax trees from Sumatra and Siam. |
| Brewer's Yeast | Vitamin B compound. |
| Butter (unsalted) | Used since early times as a cosmetic product. |
| Castor Oil | Extracted from castor beans. Strengthens hair by forming a protective film. |
| Cinnamon | Gives soap a spicy perfume and helps it to lather. |
| Citric Acid | A preservative and P.H. balancer. |

| Ingredient | Properties |
|---|---|
| Cocoa Butter | Saturated fat extracted from cocoa seeds. Suitable for body moisturising, but is too heavy for use on facial skin. |
| Coconut Oil | Adds lots of lather to soap, but is somewhat drying. Do not use on facial skin as fat molecules are too large and may clog pores. |
| Coffee | A natural deodorizer. Coffee grounds added to soap will remove kitchen odours such as fish, garlic and soap from your hands. |
| Corn Starch | A better alternative for talc. Silky and soothing in the bath tub. |
| Cottonseed Oil | A rich emollient with good keeping qualities. Useful as a carrier oil. |
| Distilled Water | Water is the single most beneficial additive for your skin. Always hydrate with pure water before applying creams. |
| Emu Oil | The closest oil to our human sebum, so emu oil has brilliant penetrating qualities. Used for centuries by the Australian Aborigines, it is now being recognised as a medical and cosmetic boon. |
| Essential Oils | See P. 58-62. |

| Ingredient | Properties |
|---|---|
| *Frankincense Powder* | Cleansing and balancing. |
| *Fuller's Earth* | A fine clay which gently pulls out impurities and firms your skin. |
| *Gelatin* | Natural thickener. Strengthens nails. |
| *Glycerin\** | * Synthetic glycerine, derived from petroleum products, may dehydrate your skin by robbing it of moisture.<br><br>The glycerine you purchase in your drug store is probably synthetic. Natural glycerine is harder to find and more expensive.<br><br>* Natural glycerine is formed as part of the saponification process, and constitutes about 25% of natural soap. It is a gentle and beneficial moisturiser. |
| *Goat's Milk* | Because goat's milk is rich and naturally homogenised, it makes wonderful creamy soap that feels like silk on your skin. |
| *Grapeseed Oil* | A gentle, versatile oil with good keeping qualities. |
| *Honey* | A traditional healer for damaged skin. Use unpasteurized, liquid honey, and do not overheat, or you will destroy the enzymes. |

| Ingredient | Properties |
|---|---|
| Jojoba Oil | Helps skin retain water. Aids in cell renewal. |
| Liquid Lecithin | A rich derivative of soy beans. Stabilises and emulsifies. |
| Lye (Sodium Hydroxide) | Reacts with fats to form soap and natural glycerine. |
| Myrrh | Fragrant gum resin from Arabia and East Africa. Used for making incense, perfume and soap. |
| Oat Flakes | Boil and strain through a nylon. The liquid makes skin silky soft. |
| Olive Oil | The main ingredient of the original Castile soap from Spain. |
| Pectin | A water-soluble carbohydrate powder or gel. Make your own by boiling apple skins. |
| Pink Clay | Naturally occurring clay, used for colour in soaps or cosmetics. |
| Pumice | The only rock that floats! A porous, soft, volcanic rock, it makes an excellent exfoliant, and does a good job of scrubbing calluses from the feet. Pumice powder can be added to soap for extra scrubbing power. |

| Ingredient | Properties |
| --- | --- |
| *Rice Flour* | A safe alternative to talc. |
| *Sea Salt* | Cleanser and exfoliant. |
| *Sesame Oil* | A bland oil with sun-screening properties. |
| *Shea Butter* | From the fruit of the karite tree. Healing for skin and hair. Helps stretch marks. |
| *Soya Oil* | A rich oil derived from Soya beans. Helpful in the healing of skin cancer spots. |
| *Spirulina* | A perfect balance of nutrients. Gives a brilliant green colour to soaps, ointments, etc. |
| *Sunflower Oil* | A good base oil. Rich in essential fatty acids. |
| *Sweet Almond Oil* | Safe and effective for care of facial skin. Synthetic version is toxic! |
| *Tea (4x)* | A teabag or a teaspoon of ioose tea, boiled in 2 cups water until the water is reduced to 1/2 cup, will enhance sun-screening properties and help to heal sunburn. The tannin in the tea has screening and curative properties. |

| Ingredient | Properties |
| --- | --- |
| *Titanium Dioxide* | A white clay pigment used widely in sunscreen lotions. Has been tested intensively for skin safety. Like most powders, it should not be inhaled. Use only cosmetic quality, coated titanium dioxide. |
| *Unsalted Butter* | One of the earliest known cosmetics. A moisturiser for body and hair. |
| *Yoghurt* | Full of natural nutrients and enzymes. |
| *Zeolite (Volcanic Clay)* | A natural clay that has the ability to perform ion exchange, to remove odours and impurities, and to filter out toxins. Leaves skin free of grease and poisons. |

# HERBAL INGREDIENTS

◆ ◆ ◆

| Herb | Properties |
|------|-----------|
| Alkanet Root | Soaked in oil, it makes deep red colouring for lip gloss. Turns purple when used in soap. |
| Annato Seeds | Yellow colouring for soap. |
| Avocado | Yields an oil rich in vitamins, minerals, and amino acids. Promotes healing. |
| Bay Leaves | Aromatic and toning. |
| Beet Powder | Natural colour for lip glosses. |
| Birch Leaves | Astringent, antiseptic. |
| Burdock | Antibacterial used for eczema and irritations. |
| Calendula Petals | From the English type of marigolds, not the South African variety. Known traditionally as a skin-healer. |
| Carrot juice | Vitamin A promotes healing and helps to remove scars. |
| Chamomile | Soothing and softening. |
| Cinnamon | Helps soap to lather and gives it a spicy perfume. |

| Herb | Properties |
| --- | --- |
| Comfrey | Healing agent containing allantoin. |
| Cornflowers | Colourful accent and natural deodorant. |
| Cucumber | Soothing and cooling, but does not keep well. |
| Dulse | Rich in iodine and minerals. |
| Elderflowers | Skin softener and soother. High in essential fatty acids. A natural deodorant. Elderberry leaves give a red dye when boiled. |
| Fennel | For sweet breath and good digestion. |
| Grape Juice | Skin softener and natural deodorant. |
| Horsetail | Used by our Native Americans for it's antiseptic and healing properties. |
| Lavender | Fragrant and acidic. A natural deodorant. |
| Lemon Juice | P.H. balancer and natural deodorant. |
| Licorice Root | Contains glycyrrhetinic acid, which works in a manner similar to cortisone. Reduces inflammation. |
| Loofah | The "skeleton" of a plant similar to zucchini. Durable and effective as a defoliant. |

| Herb | Properties |
| --- | --- |
| Nettle | Imparts body and sheen to hair. |
| Noni | A Tahitian plant that has great healing power. |
| Papaya | Contains allantoin, a skin softener. |
| Pineapple | Source of bromelain, an enzyme that "eats" dead skin cells. |
| Poppy Seeds | Used as an exfoliant in soaps or scrubs. |
| Red Clover Blossoms | Full of healing nectar. |
| Rosemary | Regenerates and tones skin, but may cause irritation if used alone. |
| Rose petals | Acid P.H.  A source of delicate perfume. |
| Sage | Made into a "soup" or facial steam, it cleanses and stimulates the skin. Also good for a dandruff rinse. |
| Soapwort Root | A natural source of saponin. |
| Spirulina | Brilliant green colour for soap or eye shadow. |
| Star Anise | Fragrant and decorative seed pods and seeds from the anise plant.  Enhances and perfumes soap. |

| Herb | Properties |
|---|---|
| *Strawberries* | Cleansing and smoothing, but inclined to cause allergies. |
| *Tansy* | Repels insects. |
| *Tomato* | Astringent and a powerful deodorant. |
| *Tumeric* | Yields a rich yellow colouring. |
| *Walnut shells* | Brown colouring. |
| *Violet leaves (blue)* | Source of a costly essential oil. Dry for use in potpourri or bath teas. |

# COST (CDN) OF SOME INGREDIENTS

◆ ◆ ◆

*These costs are approximate only (for 4oz.)*

| Ingredient | 4 oz |
|---|---|
| Chamomile flowers | $4.00 |
| Citric Acid | $4.00 |
| Comfrey Leaf | $3.75 |
| Cocoa Butter | $5.00 |
| Coconut Oil | $2.50 |
| Elderberries | $6.00 |
| Emu Oil | $18.00 |
| Frankincense Gum | $4.75 |
| Fuller's Earth | $4.00 |
| Kelp Powder | $2.00 |
| Lavender | $5.50 |
| Lemongrass | $3.00 |
| Marigold Petals | $3.50 |
| Nettle Leaf | $4.00 |

| Ingredient | 4 oz |
| --- | --- |
| Peppermint Leaf | $3.00 |
| Pink Clay | $13.00 |
| Rosehips | $2.50 |
| Rose Petals | $5.25 |
| Shea Butter | $6.00 |
| Soapwort | $7.50 |
| Spearmint | $2.50 |
| Sweet Almond Oil | $5.00 |
| Tansy flowers | $11.00 |
| Titanium Dioxide | $10.00 |
| Vanilla Beans | $6.00 |
| Volcanic Clay (Zeolite) | $4.00 |
| Witch Hazel | $4.00 |

# THINGS I DON'T USE...
## AND WHY

◆ ◆ ◆

Some of these items may work for you, but please research them very thoroughly before exposing your skin to them.

**Anything** based on petroleum or it's derivatives... because they may contain one of a whole kaleidoscope of ingredients that are potentially damaging to your skin or your system. For example, petrolatum forms a barrier that prevents the skin from taking in oxygen and emitting wastes. It is a petro-chemical and may contain carcinogens. Replace with emu oil or shea butter.

**Glycerine (manufactured).** Because it is made from petroleum and has a similar effect on your skin to that of petrolatum. The barrier effect is the reason it makes such durable bubbles.

Not to be confused with natural glycerine, which is a product of the saponification process, and constitutes about 25% of homemade soap. This is a kinder and gentler form of glycerine. Commercial soap makers remove it from their product before the process is finished, and substitute chemicals and thickeners. It is far more valuable than the soap and can be sold separately.

It is considerably more expensive than the glycerine we generally find on the drug store shelves. Replace with slippery elm or liquid lecithin.

**Borax.** An excellent emulsifier (which is why you use it with your laundry) but it is toxic. Although there is never very much of it in a recipe, even a tiny bit of poison is a bad thing, so I don't use it any more. Just leaving it out of the recipe does not seem to make much difference, so I omit it altogether.

**Lanolin.** This is wonderful stuff... if you can find a product that has not been contaminated with insecticide. As farm kids, we used to watch the sheep being 'dipped' once a year, swimming the length of a ten-foot trough and being pushed under, heads and all, by someone with a forked pole. This did not make the sheep particularly happy, but it did soak their wool with enough insecticide to kill lice and ticks for a long time. Of course at shearing time all those lovely fleeces went away for washing and processing, and the lanolin was saved. Sadly the insecticide residue was saved too, and it is very persistent stuff. So if you buy lanolin, be very careful that it has been 'decontaminated' (a difficult thing to get answers about). I think the only way to be sure would be to raise your own sheep. In the meantime, emu oil is even more effective than lanolin, although somewhat more expensive.

**Synthetic perfumes.** Chemical ingredients are blended to create illusions. They may also create allergies and damage to our systems.  The effects of essential oils are known and can be used wisely.  Not so with synthetics. User beware.

# SOURCES

### ◆ ◆ ◆

Many of the ingredients used in these recipes can be easily found in your local supermarket or health-food store. Most health-food stores are willing to order specialty items in for you if they do not carry them. In addition, there are several suppliers of herbals, essential oils and soap-making items on the internet. Shop around for your best price.

**Soap-making**: Buy supplies locally as they are bulky and you have to pay shipping charges when ordering on the internet. Lye can be found in grocery or hardware stores.

**Herbals, clays, essential oils**: You local health food store can order these for you, or you can find them on the internet. Go to your favourite search engine and type in 'soap and cosmetic supplies' for options. A supplier that I trust is www.aquariusaroma-soap.com . They have a great variety of ingredients, reasonably priced, and they also stock small containers for your creams and lotions. A bonus for U.S. shoppers, as they can take advantage of the Canadian dollar.

**Wild things:** Identify and collect such things as elderberries (blossoms and berries), wild sage, stinging nettle, horsetail and clover.

**Garden plants:**  You can grow many of the flowers and herbs you need, from calendulas to loofahs.  Plan a cosmetic garden.

Visit my web-site www.kitchencosmetics.com for more ideas and specific sourcing information.

# NOTES